GET

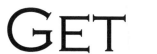 

CROCK POT RECIPES AND DIET GUIDE

SEARCHING FOR THE BEST DIET FOR YOU?
DOWNLOAD OUR FREE TOP RATED
DIETS REPORT

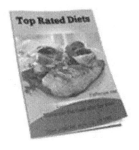

http://fitrecipe.net/FreeDietReport

BY
JESSE MORGAN

LEGAL DISCLAIMER

Thank you for either purchasing or considering a purchase of my latest book, Get Wild - Crock Pot Recipes & Diet Guide.

If you have read any of my other books, Carb Cycling: The Recipe & Diet Book, Make Ahead Meals or Blender Recipe Cookbook, you will know that I focus on diets that are healthy and use natural ingredients to help you lose weight and get fit. In the next few chapters I will help you to understand the key concepts of eating Wild.

The recipes in this book follow the guidelines setup by Abel James in his book "The Wild Diet: Get Back to Your Roots, Burn Fat, and Drop up to 20 Pounds in 40 Days". The twist with this recipe book is that you can make all of these recipes in your crock pot. Do the prep the night before, drop everything into the crock pot in the morning and fire it up. When you get home in the evening you will have a fantastic meal ready to go. We even threw in breakfast and desert recipe just to give you options.

This book is not a guide to implement the Wild Diet, you will need to purchase Abel's book and/or his information product 30 Day Fat Loss System. If you are interested in trying this diet, I definitely suggest doing both, getting his book and the fat loss system. If you are someone that has the drive and initiative to put together a system or process yourself, then you can probably just start with his book. If you want the system to support the diet, then you should definitely get his system, the cost is not much more than the book and there is so much motivational content, I think it is a no brainer. If you think about the monthly cost to do something like Weight Watchers, this solution is much cheaper and much healthier.

Please make sure to stop by our site, fitrecipe.net. You can find free content there and loads of information about the other books we have created to help you get fit and healthy while dropping those unneeded pounds. Finally if you find this book of value, please go back to the book page on Amazon and post a quick review. Reviews are so important, they help sales and help keep the books at the top of the search results in Amazon. We are constantly reinvesting revenue back into the creation of new books with the goal of helping each of you achieve your weight loss and fitness goals.

Jesse Morgan & Crew
www.fitrecipe.net

TABLE OF CONTENTS

INTRODUCTION

Why go Wild?

This book is broken into three sections:

1. Nutritional overview – Foods that will help you lose weight and get healthy.
2. Workout routines – Simple workouts you can incorporate into your schedule.
3. A fantastic set of crock pot recipes that include ingredients that fit perfectly with the Wild Diet or can just be used to create great meals for you and your family.

The goal is to return to the foods our ancestors ate before the development and creation of all of the processed foods we find in our diets today. What does your diet look like today? Are you eating processed foods, refined sugars or foods that have more chemicals in them than real ingredients?

There are three main components to succeeding with these types of diets.

1. You need to understand how bad processed foods are for

your body so that you will make the mind shift to eating real foods.

2. Change the way you shop and eat to remove processed foods from your diet.

3. Start or adjust your exercise routines to focus on full body exercises and interval training instead of endurance or general aerobic training.

REAL FOOD - NUTRITION IN A NUTSHELL

This type of diet is all about real food. Eat fresh, simple, whole foods from healthy plants and animals and avoid processed food products. Let's break this down a bit, macronutrients are nutrients needed in large amounts to provide your body with energy to maintain key functions and carry out your daily activities. Carbs, proteins, and fats are 3 essential macronutrients that are responsible for vital functions in the body.

In order for you to understand the basis of correct and healthy eating, you must know the basics of what each of these macronutrients are and what they do. If you do not, you will just fall prey to powerful marketing, which assumes you do not understand key nutrition concepts. Here's what you need to know. . .

Protein

Ideally your diet should comprise of at least 30 percent proteins, which are broken down to amino acids in the gut. Your protein intake should be at least 0.8g/kg of bodyweight, though it may vary from person to person, depending on fitness levels and activity levels. RDA recommended amounts are low, especially for the amount of amino acids you need to promote changes in the body if you are exercising. So if you are engaged in a fitness routine, it is important to consume slighter higher levels of protein from 1.5g- 2.5g/kg of bodyweight to compensate for the effects of weight training and exercise.

The need for dietary protein are the sought after amino acids. The body uses the amino acids:

- As a light/moderate energy source.
- As building blocks of DNA and muscle tissue
- As building blocks of proteins required by the body for the growth and repair of tissues, boosting immune function, and production of essential enzymes and hormones.
- As the starting material to produce other compounds.

Proteins are especially important for physically active people whose muscle tissue is in need for repair. These proteins and certain amino acids cannot be stored in the body and must be replenished every day. Proteins derived from animal sources have all the essential amino acids required by the body. During digestion, the amount of calories burned by proteins to produce energy is three to four times faster than other macronutrients, including carbohydrates and fat. The more muscle your body has, the greater the amount of calories your body burns on a daily basis (greater BMR).

Thoughts: If you wish to get more definition in your muscles or 'tone up', your diet must comprise of a significant portion of protein. Those who neglect sufficient protein intake, while still being able to lose weight with exercise and a sensible diet, are more likely to experience a higher body fat percentage and lower body weight than those who consume adequate protein amounts for their body and activity levels. You don't want to end up, 'skinny fat'.

Your best sources of protein are as follows:

White meat poultry – chicken, turkey

Seafood – tilapia, salmon, haddock, grouper, mahi, shrimp, etc.

Lean beef – lean cuts of cow (flank, eye of round, lean ground beef), venison, buffalo, NY strip, porterhouses, skirt, filet mignon, and ribeye's are still acceptable, however, just watch your portion size and weekly consumption. 4-6 oz. is all you need, not the 12-16 oz. you get served at restaurants.

Eggs – both the yolk and the white. Don't worry, it was widely regarded that the yolks caused increased cholesterol, however, that is a myth that has since been disproven by science. The AHA says you can have 1-2 whole eggs per day.

Pork tenderloin – it is the leanest cut from pork. Stay away from bacon and sausage.

Legumes – beans

Soy – tofu

Dairy – Milk, cheese, yogurt. While these do contain moderate amounts of protein, they also contain higher amounts of fat per gram or ounce than the rest on this list. Eat these sensibly and in moderation.

Carbohydrates

When creating an optimum nutrition plan for you and your family, you may find it extremely challenging to manage carbohydrate intake. After all, grains have been seen as the base of the outdated food pyramid for decades.

Unlike those misguided messages that have been ruling our lives for years, the fact is, our bodies only need a moderate amount of carbohydrates. Of course, the more physically active you are, the higher your requirement for carbohydrates becomes. Generally, your diet should comprise 35-55 percent carbohydrates.

As the main source of energy in the body, carbohydrates are broken down into glucose - the fuel needed by the body to produce energy for the heart, brain, and central nervous system.

You can find carbohydrates in most vegetables, fruits, breads, and grains. Carbohydrates can be found in the majority of foods on the shelves and in our homes. But how do we know what are good and bad carbs? In simple terms, anything that offers calories (even with small amounts) but offer NO nutritional value (ex.

Cake, cookies, white bread, soda, chips, 100 calorie snack bags) should be considered 'bad carbs.'

Your carbohydrate sources should be coming from veggies, fruits, and whole grains. It is from non-starchy vegetables that you should get the bulk of your carbohydrate intake. As these vegetables have a relatively modest carbohydrate count compared to grains and starchy veggies, they offer a greater nutrient load than the latter. You can see the list of non-starchy vs. starchy veggies on the next page:

A brief note: while it is pertinent to eat more non- starchy vegetables because they offer fewer calories and more fiber to keep us fuller longer, they also offer a much greater nutrient load from vitamins and minerals. Vitamins, minerals, potassium, antioxidants, and phytonutrients are predominantly found in the vegetables we eat. It is important to increase your vegetable consumption to increase your vitamin and mineral concentrations (termed micronutrients) in your body, this will lead to stronger immune support, enhanced blood circulation, stronger bone and joint support, and better cognitive function.

Remember, eating more carbohydrates than required by the body can sabotage your weight loss efforts, besides compromising your overall health goals. The next time you reach for that low-cal 'healthy snack', don't forget to remind yourself: carbohydrates raise blood sugar. Especially those refined processed foods that most of us have in our cabinets.

Carbohydrates can further be broken down into 4 categories:

Simple carbs are simple sugars that are digested by the body more easily and quickly. White flour, refined sugar, honey, fruit juice, fruit, chocolate, soda, jam, packaged cereals are some examples of simple carbs.

You don't have to abandon all simple sugars. Fruits are still great for you and are rich in needed micronutrients. Just be wary of the processed foods containing added sugars that cause unnecessary spikes in blood levels and additional calories. Remember, if you are following a nutritious diet, the amounts of simple sugars will be minimal anyway.

The following is a list of simple sugars you need to be aware of on food labels:

- Brown sugar
- Corn sweetener
- Corn syrup
- Dextrose
- Fructose
- Fruit juice concentrates
- Glucose
- High-fructose corn syrup
- Honey
- Invert sugar

- Lactose
- Maltose
- Malt Syrup
- Molasses
- Raw sugar
- Sucrose
- Sugar
- Syrup

While they are not all 'bad', if you consume them when the influx of sugar is not needed for extra energy exertion, it will be converted to and stored as fat. In fact, it has long been said that too much dietary fat are the causes of weight gain. However, it is becoming more and more prevalent through recent studies that processed sugar, highly consumed by Americans, is what is causing the plethora of health problems, weight gain, and other diseases.

Complex carbs are made up of three or more sugar molecules rich in vitamins, minerals, and fiber. These act as the body's fuel and don't cause blood sugar to spike as rapidly because of the longer time it take for the body to break down the molecules. They contribute considerably to long lasting energy production. Yams, Potato's, lentils, whole grains, whole grain pasta, and whole grain bread are categorized as complex carbohydrates.

Fiber may be a vision in most of our minds of Grandpa Joe eating a bowl of his favorite raisin bran cereal to help with bowel movements. While he had the right idea, you don't have to choke down dry, bland cereal. Fiber can be found naturally occurring in most vegetables as well as whole grains. You need about 15g of fiber for every 1000 calories you consume, so generally, the average person on a healthy diet should be consuming 30-35g of fiber per day. You may have also noticed on food labels that fiber is either soluble or insoluble.

Soluble fiber slows down your digestion and delays emptying of stomach contents into the lower intestines. Eating a diet rich in soluble fiber gives you a greater feeling of fullness and helps curb hunger pangs. Examples of soluble fiber are: oatmeal, oat bran, lentils, apples, oranges, pears, strawberries, nuts, flaxseeds, beans, dried peas, blueberries, psyllium, cucumbers, celery, and carrots.

Insoluble fibers have a semi-laxative effect that is great for keeping your system clean by reducing constipation. These fibers pass right through your system and increase the speed of waste through your intestines. It is mostly found in whole grains and veggies. Examples of these are whole wheat, whole grains, wheat bran, corn bran, seeds, nuts, barley, couscous, brown rice, bulgur, zucchini, celery, broccoli, cabbage, onions, tomatoes, carrots, cucumbers, green beans, dark leafy vegetables, raisins, grapes, fruit, and root vegetable skins.

Fat

Fat seems to be a dreaded word for most of us. But have you ever wondered why fat gets such a bad rap?

First, you should understand dietary fat is different than your body fat. It would seem that the lack of knowledge of nutrition scares most to think dietary fat is bad. Automatically you think, "Uh oh, I don't want any more fat on my stomach, I don't want that food if it has fat." So, is a low-fat diet a solution for all ills? Well, before answering this question, it is important to find out whether you are eating healthy fats or not.

Healthy fats include seeds, nuts, and unrefined oils and naturally occurring fats in vegetables and meats. The key lies in maintaining moderation and optimizing nutritional benefits. Experts recommend that fats and oil should suffice for at least 10–40 percent of your regular energy needs.

Though fats have earned a poor reputation for their effect on heart health and obesity, some fat is essential for health and wellbeing.

Fats:

- Help in the absorption of carotenoids and fat-soluble vitamins - A, D, E, K
- Supply essential fatty acids needed by the body, which it cannot make on its own, such as omega-3 – which is an unsaturated fat mainly found in fish.

Fats have the potential to harm as well as help our health; depending on their fatty acid composition, their nutritional value, and their condition. When used in its natural unadulterated state, fat offers optimal nutritional benefits. On the other hand, a very-low- fat diet can compromise our health and ability to lose weight.

Take a moment and look through your freezer and your cabinets, read through the ingredients of some of the products you are consuming today. I see so many people at work eating frozen pre-made lunches. Here are the ingredients from a frozen lunch for one of the popular weight loss programs:

Tortilla (Water, Enriched Flour [Bleached Wheat Flour, Niacin, Iron, Thiamine Mononitrate, Riboflavin, Folic Acid], Whole Wheat Flour, Modified Wheat Starch, Canola Oil, Wheat Gluten, Glycerine, Tomato with Pieces [Tomato Concentrate, Guar Gum], Baking Powder [Sodium Acid Pyrophosphate, Bicarbonate Soda, Cornstarch, Monocalcium Phosphate], **Hydrogenated Cottonseed Oil**, *Sugar, Salt, Granulated Garlic, Citric Acid), Cooked White Meat Chicken (White Meat Chicken, Water, Modified Potato Starch, Salt, Sodium Phosphate), Ranchero Sauce (Tomatoes [Tomatoes, Tomato Juice, Calcium Chloride, Citric Acid], Water, Chicken Base [Chicken Meat with Natural Juices, Salt, Organic Cane Juice Solids, Corn Maltodextrin, Chicken Fat,* **Yeast Extract, Natural Flavors**, *Dried Onion, Spice Extractives, Turmeric], Chili Paste [Chili Peppers, Dried Onion and Garlic, Yeast Extract, Salt, Spices, Beef Extract, Citric Acid], Roasted Tomatoes, Granulated Onion, Granulated Garlic, Jalapenos [Jalapenos, Water, Vinegar, Salt], Modified Cornstarch,* **Modified Cellulose**, *Spices, Chipotle Chili Powder], Reduced Fat Cheddar Cheese (Part Skim Milk, Cheese Culture, Salt, Enzymes, Annatto [Color]), Monterey Jack*

Cheese (Cultured Milk, Salt, Enzymes), Bell Peppers (Red, Green), Fire-Roasted Onions, Roasted Poblano Chiles, Modified Cornstarch.

Now compare that to one of the recipes in this book.

- 2 large heads escarole
- 1 small white onion, diced
- 2 cloves garlic, roughly chopped
- 4 cups beef broth
- 4 cups chicken broth
- 1/2 cup white beans, soaked overnight
- 1/2 cup chickpeas, soaked overnight
- 1 teaspoon garlic powder
- 1/2 teaspoon black pepper
- 1/2 pound meatloaf mix (beef, pork, and veal)
- 1/4 teaspoon each, salt and pepper
- 1/2 teaspoon garlic powder
- 1/2 teaspoon dried onion

Do I need to ask you which meal is the healthier alternative? OK so that is the first step to success, understanding why healthy eating is a better alternative to the way you are eating today. Next you will need to change the way you shop for foods. You may find that your grocery costs will go up changing to a healthy diet. The unfortunate reality is the cost of processed foods is much cheaper because the food companies are replacing real food ingredients with chemicals. You can walk into a food store and buy a bag of Doritos for about the same cost as one to two organic apples, or grab a bottle of soda for .99 as compared to more expensive healthier options. You have to make that decision for yourself, are you willing to put your body at risk and fail at your health and weight loss goals?

Here is a brief sample of the types of foods you should be eating:

- Fruits and Vegetables
- Strawberries, apples, cucumbers, cherry tomatoes, avocados
- Peppers, sweet potatoes, beets, spinach, broccoli
- Meats
- Ground beef, short ribs, chicken, salmon
- Dairy & Eggs
- Cheese, butter, heavy cream

Basic foods that you can find at any grocery store. You will need to focus on organic produce, wild caught fish and grass fed beef, that will increase the cost, but the quality of what you are eating is so much better for you. Would you rather eat a piece of salmon that has been feeding in its natural habitat or one that was raised in a pen being fed corn pellets? Take a look at this list of concerns regarding farm raised salmon posted at PureZing.com

1. have seven times the levels of PCB's as wild salmon
2. have 30 times the number of sea lice
3. are fed chemicals to give them color

4. are fed pellets of chicken feces, corn meal, soy, genetically modified canola oil and other fish containing concentrations of toxins

5. are administered antibiotics at higher levels than any other livestock

6. have less omega 3's due to lack of wild diet

7. are kept in small areas inhibiting movement, and causing disease

GO WILD –
GET OUT AND EXERCISE

The third area of focus is exercise. I know this might be the biggest challenge for some of you. If you want to lose weight and get fit, you need to exercise. You should always check with your doctor before starting any exercise program. Once you are cleared you should focus on two key areas; full body exercises and interval training.

Full body workouts include exercises such as squats, pushups and lunges. You can find an assortment of workouts on places like YouTube. Another great place to check is the app store for your IPhone or Android phone. If you purchase Abel's 30 Day Weight Loss program, he includes a section on exercises and a journal you can use to keep track of your workout. If you want something more structured, take a look at P90x. P90x is not for the first time exerciser, but if you have been working out regularly this program could help you get to the next level.

The second piece is interval training. Your body needs to be challenged if you want to achieve your weight loss and fitness goals. If you go out three days a week and run 3 miles at an easy pace, over time your body will adjust to that workout and will no longer be challenge by it. You may hear about endurance athletes going out for slow runs or rides to build their base, this is valid and something those athletes need to do to compete at long distances. That is not the case for the rest of us. We need to work out but the goal should be to challenge your body and force it to build new muscle. Interval training is great for this. You could go to your local gym and get on a treadmill, warm up for 10 minutes, then do 30 second bursts with 1 minute or more of recovery and then repeat that 10 times. If you like running outside or riding your bike, hill repeats are a great interval workout. Again warm up for 10 minutes and then get to a base of a hill, climb the hill as fast as you can and then recover on the way back down, do this 5 to 10 times. Please check with your doctor first before starting any new program.

Choosing Exercise Intensity: Aerobic and Anaerobic Training

Exercising at the correct intensity can help you get the most out of your physical activity — making sure you are not overdoing or underdoing it.

Intensity refers to how hard you put forth an effort to carry out a physical activity. It may vary from person to person depending on his/her strength and skill. Listen to your body's capability level , the ability to push hard during a physical activity. You will come to know the amount of physical stress you can take from exercise and what you are able to handle.

Based on your physical characteristics (age and current physical condition), you can further determine exercise intensity by the level of your heart rate (pulse). The average man or woman's pulse at rest is between 60-100 beats per minute. So to achieve fitness results, in the sense of burning more calories, your heart rate must increase during exercise.

Once your body adapts to a certain level of physical activity, you may make your activities more challenging, ensuring higher fitness levels. This is of course over the term of several months. You begin from moderate activities and progress to vigorous activities in the due course of time according to your physical condition. Once you reach new fitness levels, you can minimize or phase out exercises and activities that have become too easy and no longer offer any benefits.

Remember, challenging your body with the next level of exercise zones enhances the level of super compensation. This now brings us to a division of intensity levels and how your exercise selections further determine your fat loss and muscle building capabilities.

Aerobic Exercise

Aerobic training, in simple terms, requires you to enhance oxygen consumption at a higher than normal rate. Most common examples are jogging, running, swimming, aerobics, dance, treadmill, climbing up stairs and intense sports.

The meaning of the word aerobic is "living in air." Those exercises that demand higher use of oxygen for metabolism than normal or "lighter activities" are grouped as aerobic training.

When you undertake physical activities that go beyond the normal level and involve speed and increasingly intense movements, you begin to breathe more rapidly. This is due to a sudden increase in metabolism and fat burning which requires your lungs to supply oxygen at a higher amount and at a much faster rate.

You should try to schedule an intense aerobic activity three times-a-week at 15-20 minutes per workout with a warmup and cool-down period. Here are some of the benefits of intense aerobic activities.

- Strengthening of the muscles
- Enhancing metabolism to burn more calories
- Superior respiratory ability
- Improving efficiency and stroke volume of the heart
- Facilitating the flow of air in and out of the lungs
- Increase in red blood cells and oxygen circulation
- Reduced stress and lowering of depression
- Improved cognitive capacity
- Stimulate bone growth
- Enhanced energy molecule storage leading to improved muscle mass
- Greater endurance and mobility
- Improved use of fat and intramuscular glycogen

- Higher fitness level
- Better quality of life

Anaerobic Exercise

Intense exercises that use up oxygen faster than the body is able to replenish are known as anaerobic exercises. Muscle fibers are so intensely put to work that they use the oxygen available quickly and depend on stored carbohydrates (glycogen) to continue their task.

Sprinting, weight lifting, individual muscle-focused exercises, high-intensity interval training, powerlifting, squat, bench press, deadlift, sprinting on treadmill, etc., are examples of anaerobic training.

Anaerobic training involves very high intense and fast exercises/ workouts that puts forth maximum levels of exertion. Short bursts of strenuous activity help build your muscle fibers and endow them with higher endurance, power, strength and definition.

The rapid and exclusive use of glucose catabolism (the breakdown of glucose) during anaerobic metabolism leads to lactic acid formation. The build-up of lactic acid in muscle tissue is what causes "the burn" of your muscles. Depending on your experience level, this "burning" sensation, or tight feeling will last 30 seconds to several minutes. Don't worry, this is a good thing! As a result you feel greater fatigue and your muscles receive higher super compensation benefits in future workouts.

Aerobic and Anaerobic Exercise Complement Each Other

Aerobic exercise is a compliment to anaerobic exercise. You should combine both to accomplish a balanced fitness level.

The former acts as a stepping stone to the latter. Anaerobic work adds tone and magnifies the physical result of your aerobic exercise. Athletes begin with aerobic activity and are graduated to anaerobic activity to improve physical strength, enhance endurance, complement skill and maintain fitness levels.

If you continue with aerobic exercise alone, you may achieve the fitness level, but cannot proceed beyond that and showcase your optimal performance.

Similarly, continuing with anaerobic exercise alone puts your body into a more fatigued state and increases the production of lactic acid. You may not be able to expand the session for long because your aerobic capacity is weak. Aerobic exercise comes to your rescue here and offers an avenue to maintain the fitness level without raising the fatigue level further and becoming burnt out.

Aerobic and anaerobic are meeting points where they complement to form a person with great physical abilities. A balance between aerobic and anaerobic exercises is a must to maximize results. While the former-type of activities ensures complete workout of the body, the latter focuses on a particular muscle or part of body. Let's put this into simple terms:

Example: If you only run on the treadmill or do the elliptical at the gym at a consistent pace, you are performing aerobic exercise. This is great, and you will see an overall progression in your weight loss. However, because you are not partaking in resistance or weight training, your muscular tone, shape, and overall physical strength will not be as noticeable as someone who trains their muscles with weights. By doing aerobic exercise alone, you burn both fat and muscle.

Example 2: If you are someone who trains only with weights, the odds are you will have more strength, more muscle structure, and more shape to your body. However, your ability to uptake oxygen for long durations at a time will be minimal and your muscles may not be as defined because you are not doing enough aerobic exercises to burn fat.

The bottom line that all fitness professionals are in agreement with is . . . you MUST have a balanced routine for both cardio exercises (aerobic training) and weight lifting (anaerobic training). This is paramount for you to see massive results, and this goes for both men AND for women.

Interval Training

It is becoming increasingly accepted that shorter, more intense bouts of exercise, boost both short term and long-term exercise capacity, resulting in more efficient workouts that take a fraction of the time. A few minutes of intense activity interspersed between less intense stretches of exercise will burn excess calories all day long. Exercises can be grouped into Aerobic and Anaerobic based on the level of intensity involved. So does your notion of training revolve around working out at the same pace every day? Well, you might be losing out somewhere.

Why Interval Training

Research shows that interval training, which involves alternate periods of low and high-intensity workouts, burns more calories over a short period compared to steady-state exercise. Not only this, it also increases fitness and conditioning levels.

During an interval training session, you can expect many physiological changes. This may include boost in cardiovascular efficiency and improved tolerance to the increase in lactic acid. You benefit in more ways than one from these changes, including greater speed, improved performance, and higher endurance.

Alternating short bursts of high-intensity exercise with short, less intense activity will help avoid injuries often resulting from repetitive overuse of muscles. These types of injuries are more common for endurance athletes. A consistent pace of high-intensity activity is difficult to maintain. However, intervals allow you to raise training intensity without burn-out. Such type of interval training is a great way to add cross training to your workout regimen.

Interval training helps burn more calories. According to the American College of Sports Medicine, short high intensity exercise burns more calories in a shorter amount of time than long, slow endurance exercise. Interval training utilizes the aerobic and anaerobic body system. While the aerobic system uses oxygen to convert carbohydrates and fat into energy that allows you to practice for a longer duration, the anaerobic system uses energy in the form of glycogen from carbohydrates to support short, intense activities.

Sample Interval Workouts

You can pick a single routine and perform it the indicated amount of days I have specified per week OR you can mix and match all the routines as long as you get 3-5 workouts in per week.

15 MINUTE BODY WEIGHT RESISTANCE WORKOUT	
BEGINNER	• Perform 7 rounds of the following exercises • Start with 5 reps, add an additional 2 reps each round. • Rest 45 seconds between rounds
EXERCISES	1. Body Weight Squat 2. Dips (use sturdy surface that is lower to the ground. Edge of bed, chair, or couch) 3. Pushups (use edge of bed or table to elevate yourself if on the floor becomes too difficult) 4. Superman's (YouTube this exercise)

15 MINUTE BODY WEIGHT INTERVALS CARDIO/RESISTANCE

INTERMEDIATE	• Perform each exercise for 20 seconds then rest for 10 seconds, then repeat • Continue this pattern NON-STOP for the entire 15 min • Each individual exercise will be performed 4 times • 8 total exercises
EXERCISES	1. Jog in place 2. Jumping Jacks 3. Squat Jump (YouTube this) 4. Split stance squat (2 times on each leg) (YouTube this as well) 5. Push ups 6. Crunches 7. Planks 8. Side plank (2 times each side)

15 MIN BODY WEIGHT INTERVALS CARDIO/RESISTANCE

HARD	• Perform Each exercise for 20 seconds then rest for 10 seconds • Continue this NON-STOP for 15 min • Each exercise will be performed 4 times • 8 total exercises • Perform 3-5 times per week
EXERCISES	1. High Knees 2. Pop squats 3. Spiderman Push-ups 4. Burpees 5. Mountain Climbers 6. Switch kicks 7. Squat position hold 8. Side plank rotations

30 MIN BODY WEIGHT INTERVALS

HARD	• Perform each exercise for 20 seconds and lightly jog in place for 20 seconds
	• There are 6 intense Exercises combined with 6 bouts of jogging per each round. Each round lasts 4 min
	• After all 6 Intense exercises are complete, rest for 1 – 1 ½ min
	• Repeat for total of 6 rounds
	• Perform 3 times per week
EXERCISES	1. Jog in Place – 20 sec
	2. #1 Jumping Jacks – 20 seconds Jog in Place – 20 sec
	3. #2 Squat Jumps – 20 seconds Jog in Place – 20 sec
	4. #3 Mountain Climbers – 20 seconds Jog in Place – 20 sec
	5. #4 Burpees – 20 seconds Jog in Place – 20 sec
	6. #5 Ski Downs – 20 seconds Jog in Place – 20 sec
	7. #6 High Knees – 20 seconds

40 MIN WEIGHT TRAINING INTERVALS

WORKOUT A	• 3 series of weighted exercises
	• 3 rounds for EACH series
	• Complete 1 round within 2 minutes (keep track of this)
	• Rest 1 minute between rounds
	• This will take 27min – 40 min depending on your rest times
	• Perform this workout 2-3 times per week

EXERCISES	**REPS**
Series 1 Incline Dumbbell press Reverse lunge hold dumbbells Hammer curls	12-15 10 each leg (1 leg at time) 12-15
Series 2 Seated Cable Row Dumbbell Goblet Squat Standing Barbell press	12-15 12-15 12-15
Series 3 Lat Pulldown Kettle Bell swing Tricep Rope Push Down	12-15 12-15 12-15

40 MIN WEIGHT TRAINING INTERVALS

WORKOUT B	• 3 series of weighted exercises
	• 3 rounds for EACH series
	• Complete 1 round within 2 minutes (keep track of this)
	• Rest 1 minute between rounds
	• This will take 27min – 40 min depending on your rest times
	• Perform this workout 2-3 times per week

EXERCISES	**REPS**
Series 1 *Flat barbell press Split squat* *Seated palms up dumbbell curls*	12-15 12 each leg 12-15
Series 2 *Barbell deadlift* *Seated Overhead dumbbell press* *Standing lateral raises*	12-15 12-15 12-15
Series 3 *Stiff arm Lat Pulldown* *Kettle Bell or dumbbell swing Tricep* *Rope overhead extensions*	12-15 12-15 12-15

FUN FITNESS FOR MOTIVATION

Experts believe that fun and fitness are correlated – you benefit the most from a fitness workout when you are having fun. Do an exercise you enjoy. If you don't enjoy doing it, you'll find one excuse or the other not to do it. Soon you will come up with an excuse of pain or boredom.

Contrarily, when an exercise seems fun to you, you're likely to find enjoyment in it, which is more likely to distract your attention from the "pain" of working out. You will have the willpower to work out longer.

Undoubtedly, fun is the most important "ingredient" when it comes to working out. It can help keep you motivated, focused, and energetic.

It is important to find what fun is for you and what interests you. Make the commitment to doing it for the long haul and set short-term and long-term goals.

Simply going through the motions is not going to pay you much dividends. It is guaranteed to be ineffective.

Let your fitness regimen be invigorating and enjoyable. Don't think of it as a burden. Don't make it compulsory merely for the sake of doing. Find enjoyment in it to make it productive. Do it for a healthy life. Exercise is crucial to stay mentally and spiritually healthy as well as physical fit.

Fitness may be fun if you work out in a group. Choose a fitness partner. Why not ask a like-minded friend or even your partner to accompany you as a fitness mate? If you are not able to convince your partner or a friend, try to find people with similar fitness goals. Make your fitness social.

- Enjoy the therapy of fitness.
- Appreciate the beauty of the world if you are working out in the open.
- Have fun and feel good. Let the motivation to stay fit keep you working out toward being healthy.
- Don't feel bad about your body, as this may only force you into engaging in a strenuous exercise that you do not enjoy. This will mean that you won't be able to maintain your exercise regimen for long, because you do not enjoy it or find no pleasure doing it.
- Expect ups and downs when you start working out. There may be days when you don't feel good to work out. It's absolutely ok to skip. Don't be discouraged with it. It happens with almost everyone, including myself!

- Instead of spending time and energy on feeling guilty of having missed your fitness regimen, focus on what it'll take to resume working out again. With such mind-set, when you rekindle your motivation and resume your fitness regimen, you'll be surprised to see how quickly it will begin to feel natural. Get started again and gradually reclaim your routine and build up to your momentum.

CROCK POT GET WILD RECIPES

HONEY BARBECUE CHICKEN WINGS

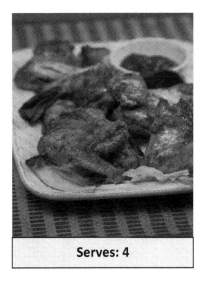

Serves: 4

INGREDIENTS:

- ➤ 4 pounds fresh chicken wings
- ➤ 1/4 cup tomato paste
- ➤ 2 tablespoons raw honey
- ➤ 2 tablespoons blackstrap molasses
- ➤ 3 tablespoons raw apple cider vinegar
- ➤ 2 cloves garlic, minced
- ➤ 1 teaspoon dried onion
- ➤ 1 teaspoon paprika
- ➤ 1/2 teaspoon ground mustard
- ➤ 1/2 teaspoon oregano
- ➤ 1/2 teaspoon pepper
- ➤ 1/4 teaspoon cayenne pepper

INSTRUCTIONS:

Add all ingredients, except for chicken wings into a small saucepan and cook over low heat, stirring often for five minutes. Set aside about 1/4 cup of sauce for dipping later. Add your chicken wings to your slow cooker and pour over the remaining barbecue sauce. Cook wings on low for 6 hours. Preheat your oven to broil, lay the wings flat onto a baking sheet and broil about 1 minute on each side, until crispy. Use the leftover sauce for dipping if you'd like.

NUTRITION:

Calories: 322	Fat: 18g	Carbs: 18g	Protein: 22g

Galumpkis (Stuffed Cabbage)

Serves: 4

Ingredients:

- ➢ 1 large head green cabbage
- ➢ 1 pound lean ground beef
- ➢ 1 small white onion, minced
- ➢ 2 cloves garlic, minced
- ➢ 1/2 green bell pepper, diced
- ➢ 1 cup cauliflower rice*
- ➢ 1/2 teaspoon each, salt and pepper
- ➢ 2 tablespoons sauce

For sauce:

- ➢ 1 pint cherry tomatoes
- ➢ 1/4 cup water
- ➢ 1/2 teaspoon garlic powder
- ➢ 1/2 teaspoon oregano

Instructions:

Remove stem from cabbage and pull leaves apart. Pick out 12 large leaves. Lay the leaves into a microwave safe dish, add a 1/2 inch of water, cover with plastic wrap and then microwave on high for two minutes. Remove the cabbage from the microwave and allow to cool while you prepare the meat mixture. In a large bowl, add ground beef, onion, garlic, bell pepper, cauliflower rice, salt and pepper, mix well. Add cherry tomatoes, water, garlic powder, and oregano to a blender or food processor and blend until a smooth sauce forms, about 45 seconds. Add two tablespoons of the sauce to the meat mixture, stir well and then spoon an equal size mixture into each cabbage leaf. Wrap the the leaves up and then lay them gently into the crockpot. Pour over all of the sauce mixture, making sure it coats each roll evenly and then cook on low for 8 hours, enjoy!

* Cauliflower rice: Use a cheese shredder or food processor to grate or process the cauliflower into rice size pieces.

NUTRITION:

Calories: 226	Fat: 8g	Carbs: 12g	Protein: 26g

LOWER CARB BEEF STEW

Serves: 4

INGREDIENTS

- ➢ 1 pound stew meat, cut into 1" cubes
- ➢ 2 tablespoons coconut or brown rice flour
- ➢ 1 small white onion, diced
- ➢ 2 cloves garlic, minced
- ➢ 6 ribs celery, sliced into 1" pieces
- ➢ 1 pound baby carrots
- ➢ 3 large parsnips, peeled and cut into bit sized pieces
- ➢ 8 ounces white button mushrooms, halved
- ➢ 1 teaspoon garlic powder
- ➢ 1 teaspoon paprika
- ➢ 1/2 teaspoon each, salt and pepper
- ➢ 2 bay leaves
- ➢ 2 cups beef broth

INSTRUCTIONS:

Add the stewing meat to your crock pot and sprinkle the flour over the meat. Stir gently to ensure each piece is coated. Add vegetables, sprinkle over seasonings, pour over the beef broth and then cook on high for 6 hours. Remove bay leaves and enjoy!

NUTRITION:

Calories: 379	Fat: 19g	Carbs: 22g	Protein: 27g

EASY LEMON DILL SALMON

Serves: 2

INGREDIENTS:

- ➢ 2 pieces of foil, 1 foot long
- ➢ 2, 6 ounce salmon filets (wild caught if possible)
- ➢ 1 bunch fresh dill (or 1 tablespoon dried dill weed)
- ➢ 1 large lemon, sliced into 6 thin slices
- ➢ 1/2 teaspoon each, salt and pepper

INSTRUCTIONS:

Lay each piece of foil flat on your countertop. Rinse the salmon and then lay each piece on their own sheet of tinfoil. Lay sprigs of fresh dill over each filet, or sprinkle with dried dill, top each filet with three slices of lemon, sprinkle with salt and pepper. Pull up the edges of the foil and crimp to secure them, gently transfer each packet to the crockpot. Cook on low for about three hours, until flakey. Once cooked, allow to cool and enjoy with a side of steamed vegetables.

NUTRITION:

Calories: 234	Fat: 10g	Carbs: 1g	Protein: 33g

CROCK POT ARTICHOKES

Serves: 4

INGREDIENTS:

- ➤ 4 x-large artichokes (look for the largest ones you can find)
- ➤ 1 cup chicken stock
- ➤ 2 cloves garlic, minced
- ➤ Juice of 1 lemon
- ➤ 2 tablespoons grass-fed butter at room temperature
- ➤ 1/4 teaspoon pepper

INSTRUCTIONS:

Cut the stems off of the artichokes, ensuring that the ends are straight so they will be able to stand easily. Slice the top 1" of the artichokes off. Place all artichokes upwards in the crockpot (if there is any extra space which causes them to fall, simply fill the space with a ball of tinfoil). Pour chicken stock into the bottom of the crock pot. In a small bowl, add garlic, lemon juice, butter, and pepper, mix well and then use a brush to brush the butter mixture on top of each artichoke. Cover your crockpot and cook until the artichokes are soft, about 3 1/2 hours. To enjoy artichokes, simply pull off the leaves and enjoy the meat at the bottom of each leaf. Once all leaves are removed, you can cut away the the pitch and enjoy the choke which is hidden in the middle.

NUTRITION:

Calories: 115	Fat: 6g	Carbs: 6g	Protein: 4g

BEAN-LESS CHILI

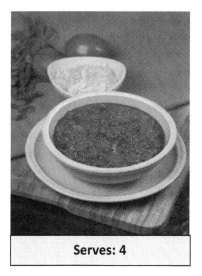

Serves: 4

INGREDIENTS:

- ➢ 1 pound lean ground beef
- ➢ 3 cloves garlic, minced
- ➢ 1 vadalia onion, diced
- ➢ 1 green bell pepper, diced
- ➢ 4 ribs celery, sliced into 1/2" pieces
- ➢ 2 beefsteak tomatoes, diced
- ➢ 1 can organic tomato paste such as Mur Glen

- ➢ 1 tablespoon garlic powder
- ➢ 2 tablespoons chili powder
- ➢ 1 teaspoon paprika
- ➢ 1 teaspoon dried oregano
- ➢ 1/2 teaspoon dried basil
- ➢ 1/2 teaspoon each, salt and pepper
- ➢ 1/4 teaspoon cayenne pepper
- ➢ Optional Toppings:
- ➢ Fresh sliced avocado
- ➢ Fresh cilantro
- ➢ Chopped chives or green onions
- ➢ Fresh diced tomatoes

INSTRUCTIONS:

Add all chili ingredients into a crock pot and mix well to ensure everything is incorporated. Cook on low for 8 hours. Ladle chili into bowls, top with optional toppings and enjoy!

NUTRITION (ASSUMING NO OPTIONAL TOPPINGS)

Calories: 215	Fat: 5g	Carbs: 18g	Protein: 24g

BERRY CRUMBLE

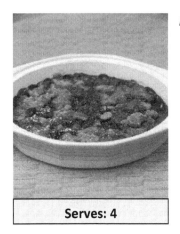

Serves: 4

INGREDIENTS:

- ➢ 1 pound fresh or frozen mixed berries
- ➢ 2 tablespoons lemon juice
- ➢ 1/2 cup almond flour
- ➢ 2 tablespoons coconut flour
- ➢ 1/4 cup chopped walnuts
- ➢ 2 teaspoons cinnamon
- ➢ 1/2 teaspoon nutmeg
- ➢ 2 tablespoons coconut oil
- ➢ 2 tablespoons raw honey

INSTRUCTIONS:

Spray your slow cooker with nonstick spray. Pour in your fresh and frozen berries, sprinkle over lemon juice, mix gently and spread out the berries so they form an even layer on the bottom. Add all remaining ingredients to a small bowl and mix well until you get a crumbly and cohesive mixture. Evenly pour your topping oven the berries, cover your slow cooker and cook on high for 1 hour and 30 minutes. Enjoy with a dollop of fresh whipped cream. This is a perfect dessert to throw in you slow cooker before dinner and have warm and ready to serve later on for dessert.

NUTRITION:

Calories: 265	Fat: 17g	Carbs: 27g	Protein: 5g

ITALIAN WEDDING SOUP

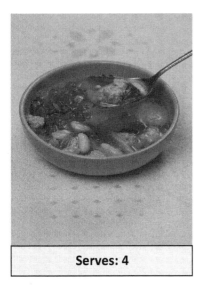

Serves: 4

INGREDIENTS:

- ➢ 2 large heads escarole
- ➢ 1 small white onion, diced
- ➢ 2 cloves garlic, roughly chopped
- ➢ 4 cups beef broth
- ➢ 4 cups chicken broth
- ➢ 1/2 cup white beans, soaked overnight
- ➢ 1/2 cup chickpeas, soaked overnight
- ➢ 1 teaspoon garlic powder
- ➢ 1/2 teaspoon black pepper
- ➢ 1/2 pound meatloaf mix (beef, pork, and veal)
- ➢ 1/4 teaspoon each, salt and pepper
- ➢ 1/2 teaspoon garlic powder
- ➢ 1/2 teaspoon dried onion

INSTRUCTIONS:

Rinse escarole really well to ensure you get all of the dirt off of it. Roughly chop escarole and then transfer to your slow cooker. Sprinkle diced onion on top of the escarole, add garlic, beef and chicken broth, soaked white beans and chickpeas, 1 teaspoon garlic powder and 1/2 teaspoon black pepper. In a medium bowl, add meatloaf mix, salt, pepper, garlic powder, and onion and mix well. Form into small, bite-sized meatballs and lay them on top of the escarole. Place the lid on your slow cooker and cook on low for 6-8 hours, enjoy!

NUTRITION:

Calories: 292	Fat: 18g	Carbs: 16g	Protein: 14g

SESAME CHICKEN

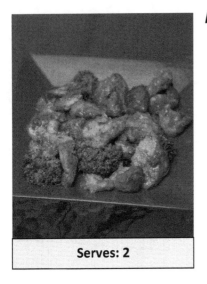

Serves: 2

INGREDIENTS:

- ➢ 2, 6 ounce boneless, skinless organic chicken breasts
- ➢ 2 tablespoons coconut or brown rice flour
- ➢ 1 tablespoon arrowroot powder
- ➢ 2 cloves garlic, minced
- ➢ 1 teaspoon dried onion flakes
- ➢ 2 teaspoons sesame seeds
- ➢ 1 tablespoon raw honey
- ➢ 3 tablespoons coconut aminos
- ➢ 1/2 teaspoon black pepper
- ➢ 2 cups fresh broccoli florets

INSTRUCTIONS:

Slice chicken into very thin pieces and then place in your crockpot. Sprinkle over the flour and arrowroot powder and then gently stir the chicken to ensure each piece is coated. In a small bowl, combine garlic, dried onion, sesame seeds, honey, coconut aminos, and black pepper and stir until you have a cohesive mixture. Pour the sesame mixture over the chicken, lay the broccoli on top, place the lid on your slow cooker and cook on high for 2 hours. Reduce heat to low and cook for an additional 2 hours or until you are ready to eat. Enjoy alone or over a bed of steamed cauliflower rice.

Nutrition:

Calories: 327	Fat: 8g	Carbs: 25g	Protein: 35g

MEATBALLS IN HOMEMADE SAUCE

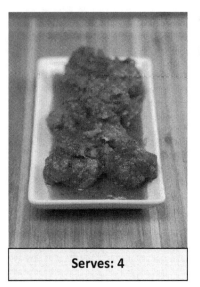

Serves: 4

INGREDIENTS:

For the Meatballs:
- ➤ 1 pound 93% lean ground beef
- ➤ 1/4 cup coconut or brown rice flour
- ➤ 1/2 cup grated white onion
- ➤ 2 cloves garlic, minced
- ➤ 1 large egg
- ➤ 1 teaspoon garlic powder
- ➤ 2 teaspoons Italian seasonings
- ➤ 1/2 teaspoon each, salt and pepper

For the Sauce:
- ➤ 1, 28 ounce can tomato puree
- ➤ 1, 14.5 ounce can diced tomatoes
- ➤ 1 tablespoon garlic powder
- ➤ 1 tablespoon dried onion
- ➤ 1 tablespoon Italian seasonings
- ➤ 1/2 teaspoon pepper
- ➤ 1/4 cup grated parmesan cheese

INSTRUCTIONS:

Add all meatball ingredients to a large mixing bowl and mix well, using your hands. Form into medium-sized balls and lay down into your crockpot. Open your two cans of tomatoes and pour them over the meatballs. Sprinkle the seasonings and parmesan cheese over the meatballs. Cover your crockpot and cook on low for 6-8 hours, stir before serving and enjoy!

NUTRITION:

Calories: 378	Fat: 12g	Carbs: 30g	Protein: 34g

GARLIC CHICKEN THIGHS

Serves: 4

INGREDIENTS:

- ➤ 8 organic, skinless chicken thighs
- ➤ 1/4 cup coconut aminos
- ➤ 2 tablespoons raw honey
- ➤ 1/4 cup tomato paste
- ➤ 4 cloves garlic, minced
- ➤ 1 teaspoon onion powder
- ➤ 1 teaspoon dried oregano
- ➤ 1 tablespoon dried parsley
- ➤ 1/2 teaspoon each, salt and pepper

INSTRUCTIONS:

Rinse your chicken thighs and lay them down in your slow cooker. Add all remaining ingredients to a mixing bowl and whisk until everything is smoothly incorporated. Pour garlic mixture over the chicken thighs, place lid on your slow cooker, and cook on high for 4 hours, enjoy! (You can also cook for 6 hours on low)

NUTRITION:

Calories: 261	Fat: 7g	Carbs: 15g	Protein: 34g

BLACK BEAN SOUP

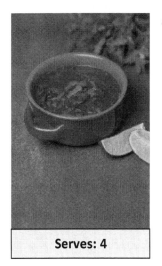

Serves: 4

INGREDIENTS:

- ➤ 2 cup dried black beans, soaked overnight
- ➤ 4 cups chicken or vegetable broth
- ➤ 2 cups water
- ➤ 1 green pepper, chopped
- ➤ 1 large white onion, diced
- ➤ 2 jalapeño peppers, seeds removed and diced
- ➤ 2 cloves garlic, minced
- ➤ 1, 14.5 ounce can diced tomatoes
- ➤ 1/2 cup raw apple cider vinegar
- ➤ 1/2-1 cup fresh cilantro, chopped
- ➤ 1 tablespoon garlic powder
- ➤ 1 tablespoon cumin
- ➤ 2 teaspoons chili powder
- ➤ 1/2 teaspoon each, salt and pepper

INSTRUCTIONS:

Add all ingredients into your slow cooker and mix to combine. Cook on high for 5-6 hours and enjoy topped with additional fresh cilantro!

NUTRITION:

Calories: 206	Fat: 0g	Carbs: 58g	Protein: 20g

CHICKEN SOUP WITH WILD RICE

Serves: 4

INGREDIENTS:

- ➢ 2, 6 ounce boneless, skinless chicken breasts
- ➢ 4 cups chicken broth
- ➢ 1/2 cup whole grain brown rice
- ➢ 1/2 cup wild rice
- ➢ 2 cups water
- ➢ 1 small white onion, diced
- ➢ 4 large carrots, sliced into 1/2" rounds
- ➢ 4 ribs celery, slice into 1/2" pieces
- ➢ 1 tablespoon dried dill weed
- ➢ 1/2 teaspoon black pepper

INSTRUCTIONS:

Slice your chicken breasts into bite-sized cubes and transfer them to your slow cooker. Pour the broth and water over the chicken and then stir in the brown and wild rice. Add the vegetables and seasonings and then cover. Cook on high heat until the chicken starts to fall apart, about 4-6 hours.

NUTRITION:

Calories: 196	Fat: 3g	Carbs: 22g	Protein: 20g

CAJUN SHRIMP

Serves: 4

INGREDIENTS:

- ➢ 2 tablespoons grass-fed butter
- ➢ 2 tablespoons fresh lemon juice
- ➢ 2 tablespoons coconut aminos
- ➢ 2 cloves garlic, minced
- ➢ 1 pound easy peel, deveined shrimp, peels left on
- ➢ 1 tablespoon cajun seasonings
- ➢ 1/2 teaspoon red pepper flakes

INSTRUCTIONS:

Add butter, lemon juice, coconut aminos, and garlic to your slow cooker and turn onto high. Allow your slow cooker to heat up. You will know it is hot when the butter has melted (this should take about 20 minutes). Once hot, add in shrimp, Cajun seasonings, and red pepper flakes. Stir to coat shrimp. Place the lid on the slow cooker and cook for 20 minutes. Stir and then cook for another 5-10 minutes, until the shrimp are opaque. Enjoy!

NUTRITION:

Calories: 179	Fat: 7g	Carbs: 2g	Protein: 23g

SAUSAGE, PEPPERS, AND ONIONS

Serves: 4

INGREDIENTS:

- ➤ 1 pound nitrate-free Italian sausage
- ➤ 1 green pepper, sliced into 1/2" strips
- ➤ 1 red pepper, sliced into 1/2" strips
- ➤ 2 large white onions, sliced thin
- ➤ 2 cloves garlic, minced
- ➤ 1/2 teaspoon each, salt and pepper

INSTRUCTIONS:

Lay sausage links onto the bottom of your slow cooker. Spread the sliced peppers and onions over the sausage. Add the garlic and sprinkle over the salt and pepper. Place the lid on your slow cooker and cook on high for 4 hours, enjoy!

NUTRITION:

Calories: 300	Fat: 21g	Carbs: 13g	Protein: 14g

JALAPEÑO PULLED PORK

Serves: 4

INGREDIENTS:

➤ 1 1/2 pounds lean pork loin
➤ 2 jalapeño peppers, seeds removed
➤ 1 medium Vidalia onion, diced
➤ 2 cloves garlic, minced
➤ 1/4 cup tomato paste
➤ 2 tablespoon blackstrap molases
➤ 3 tablespoons apple cider vinegar
➤ 1 tablespoon chili powder
➤ 2 teaspoons paprika
➤ 2 teaspoons garlic powder
➤ 1 teaspoon mustard powder
➤ 1/2 teaspoon cayenne pepper
➤ 1/2 teaspoon each salt and pepper

INSTRUCTIONS:

Place the pork loin, jalapeño peppers, and diced onion into your slow cooker. In a small bowl, add all remaining ingredients and mix well. Pour your sauce over the pork loin, cover your pot and cook on high for 4-5 hours. Use two forks to pull your pork apart, enjoy!

NUTRITION:

Calories: 249	Fat: 7g	Carbs: 13g	Protein: 36g

Chicken Cacciatore

Serves: 4

INGREDIENTS:

- ➢ 2, 6 ounce boneless, skinless chicken breasts
- ➢ 1, 28 ounce can crushed tomatoes
- ➢ 1, 28 ounce can diced or plum tomatoes
- ➢ 1 green pepper, sliced into 1/2" strips
- ➢ 1, 8 ounce package button mushrooms, sliced
- ➢ 1 tablespoon garlic powder
- ➢ 1 tablespoon Italian seasonings
- ➢ 1/2 teaspoon red pepper flakes
- ➢ 1/2 teaspoon each, salt and pepper

INSTRUCTIONS:

Add all ingredients to your slow cooker. Cover and cook for 4 hours on high, then keep on low until ready to serve, enjoy!

NUTRITION:

| Calories: 243 | Fat: 4g | Carbs: 27g | Protein: 23g |

LOW-CARB PANCAKES

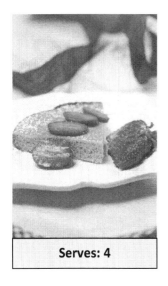

Serves: 4

INGREDIENTS:

> ➢ 3/4 cup low-fat cottage cheese
> ➢ 2 eggs
> ➢ 1 tablespoon coconut oil
> ➢ 1 teaspoon vanilla extract
> ➢ 1/4 cup almond milk
> ➢ 1 cup coconut flour
> ➢ 1/2 teaspoon baking soda
> ➢ 1 teaspoon stevia powder

OPTIONAL: sliced strawberries or pure maple syrup for topping

INSTRUCTIONS:

Add the first five ingredients to a food processor and process for 30 seconds. Add flour, baking soda and stevia to the processor and pulse until combined, about 15 seconds. Spray your slow cooker well with nonstick cooking spray and then pour your batter in, ensuring there is an even layer across. Turn your slow cooker on high, cover, and cook for 1 hour. After an hour, turn your slow cooker off and allow your pancake to cool before removing it with a rubber spatula. Slice into 6 portions and enjoy!

NUTRITION:

Calories: 150	Fat: 7g	Carbs: 13g	Protein: 8.5g

SHRIMP AND SAUSAGE GUMBO

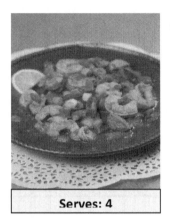

Serves: 4

INGREDIENTS:

> 1 large white onion, diced
> 6 ribs celery, sliced into 1/2" pieces
> 1 green bell pepper, chopped into 1/2" pieces
> 1, 28 ounce can, plum tomatoes
> 1 cup chicken broth
> 4 cloves garlic, minced
> 2 teaspoons ground thyme
> 1/2 teaspoon each, salt and pepper
> 1 tablespoon paprika
> 1 teaspoon cayenne pepper
> Optional: 1 tablespoon file powder
> 6 ounces andouille sausage, sliced into 1/2-1" pieces
> 1 pound large shrimp, peeled and deveined with tails removed

INSTRUCTIONS:

Add all ingredients except the sausage and shrimp into your slow cooker and mix well to ensure the herbs are evenly distributed. Add in the sausage, cover and cook on low for 6-8 hours. Turn your slow cooker on high, stir in your shrimp and cook for 30-45 minutes, until desired doneness. Enjoy as is or over brown rice.

NUTRITION:

| Calories: 320 | Fat: 13g | Carbs: 16g | Protein: 29g |

BLACK PEPPER FLANK STEAK

Serves: 4

INGREDIENTS:

- ➢ 2 cloves garlic, minced
- ➢ 2 tablespoons coconut aminos
- ➢ 1 tablespoon olive oil
- ➢ 1 tablespoon blackstrap molases
- ➢ 1 tablespoon ground black pepper
- ➢ 1/2 teaspoon salt
- ➢ 1 1/2 pounds lean flank steak

INSTRUCTIONS:

Add garlic, coconut amines, olive oil, molasses, pepper, and salt into a small bowl and mix to combine. Place the flank steak onto a plate and rub each side with the pepper mixture. Transfer your flank steak to your crock pot and cook for 6-8 hours on high. Remove steak from your slow cooker and slice, enjoy!

NUTRITION:

Calories: 413	Fat: 21g	Carbs: 5g	Protein: 47g

BALSAMIC CHICKEN WITH TOMATOES

Serves: 2

INGREDIENTS:

- ➢ 2, 6 ounce boneless, skinless chicken breasts
- ➢ 4 large roma tomatoes, diced
- ➢ 2 tablespoons balsamic vinegar
- ➢ 2 cloves garlic, minced
- ➢ 1/2 teaspoon each, salt and pepper

INSTRUCTIONS:

Slice chicken breasts in half and lay them into your slow cooker. Add diced tomatoes, vinegar, garlic, salt and pepper to a bowl and mix well. Pour over the chicken, cover, and cook for 4 hours on high, enjoy!

NUTRITION:

Calories: 216	Fat: 9g	Carbs: 9g	Protein: 34g

BEEF TERIYAKI WITH PEA PODS

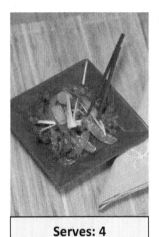

Serves: 4

INGREDIENTS:

- ➤ 2 tablespoons coconut aminos
- ➤ 1 tablespoon rice wine vinegar
- ➤ 1 tablespoon blackstrap molasses
- ➤ 2 cloves garlic, minced
- ➤ 1 tablespoon arrowroot powder
- ➤ 1 teaspoon dried ground ginger
- ➤ 1 teaspoon garlic powder
- ➤ 1 teaspoon red pepper flakes
- ➤ 1/2 teaspoon black pepper
- ➤ 1 pound lean beef, such as skirt steak, sliced into thin strips
- ➤ 1/2 pound fresh sugar-snap peas
- ➤ 2 large carrots, sliced into 1/2" pieces

INSTRUCTIONS:

Add all ingredients except for beef and pea pods to a large bowl and mix well. Add your beef and stir to ensure each piece is evenly coated. Pour into your slow cook and then add the pea pods on top. Cover and cook on high for 1 1/2 hours, enjoy alone or over brown rice.

NUTRITION:

Calories: 231	Fat: 9g	Carbs: 11g	Protein: 26g

BAKED BEANS

Serves: 6

INGREDIENTS:

- 4 slices nitrate free thick-sliced bacon, cut into 1" pieces
- 1 large white onion, diced
- 2 cups navy beans, soaked overnight and drained
- 1/2 cup blackstrap molases
- 1 can tomato paste
- 2 teaspoons stevia
- 1 teaspoon ground mustard powder
- 1 teaspoon each, salt and pepper

INSTRUCTIONS:

Lay bacon pieces into the bottom of your slow cooker and pour in the diced onion and soaked beans. In a small bowl, mix the molasses, tomato paste, stevia, mustard powder, and salt and pepper. Pour mixture over the beans. Pour over three cups of warm water, place on the lid and then cook on high for six hours, enjoy!

NUTRITION:

| Calories: 245 | Fat: 5g | Carbs: 45g | Protein: 14g |

SLOW COOKED RIBS

Serves: 4

INGREDIENTS:

- ➢ 3 pounds baby back ribs, trimmed
- ➢ 1/2 cup tomato paste
- ➢ 1/4 cup water
- ➢ 1/4 cup blackstrap molases
- ➢ 2 tablespoons raw apple cider vinegar
- ➢ 1 teaspoon mustard powder
- ➢ 1 teaspoon garlic powder
- ➢ 1 teaspoon paprika
- ➢ 1/4 teaspoon cayenne pepper
- ➢ 1/2 teaspoon each, salt and pepper

INSTRUCTIONS:

Place ribs laying flat into your slow cooker. Add all remaining ingredients to a bowl and mix well. Set aside 1/4 cup of the sauce and pour the rest over the ribs, place on lid, and cook on low for 8 hours. Remove ribs from slow cooker, baste with the barbecue sauce you set aside and enjoy!

NUTRITION:

Calories: 634	Fat: 43g	Carbs: 16g	Protein: 42g

KALE AND SWEET POTATO SOUP

Serves: 4

INGREDIENTS:

- ➤ 1 head kale, washed and chopped
- ➤ 2 large sweet potatoes, peeled and cut into 1" cubes
- ➤ 1/2 cup white onion, diced
- ➤ 2 cloves garlic, minced
- ➤ 1/2 cup quinoa
- ➤ 1 cup red beans, soaked overnight
- ➤ 8 cups chicken broth
- ➤ 1 tablespoons Italian seasonings
- ➤ 2 teaspoons garlic powder
- ➤ 1/2 teaspoon red pepper flakes
- ➤ 1/2 teaspoon each salt and pepper

INSTRUCTIONS:

Add all ingredients to your slow cooker and mix. Cover and cook on high for 4-6 hours, serve and enjoy!

NUTRITION:

Calories: 290	Fat: 1g	Carbs: 69g	Protein: 16g

CREAMY CHICKEN WITH MUSHROOMS

Serves: 4

INGREDIENTS:

- ➤ 4, 6 ounce boneless, skinless chicken breasts
- ➤ 8 ounces baby bella mushrooms, sliced
- ➤ 1 large white onion, diced
- ➤ 2 cloves garlic, minced
- ➤ 1 cup chicken broth
- ➤ 1/4 cup heavy cream
- ➤ 2 tablespoons arrowroot powder
- ➤ 1 teaspoon ground thyme
- ➤ 1/4 teaspoon each, salt and pepper

INSTRUCTIONS:

Slice chicken breasts in half and then lay into crock pot. Add sliced mushrooms, diced onion, and minced garlic on top of the chicken breasts. In a small bowl, mix chicken broth, heavy cream, arrowroot powder, and seasonings and then pour into crock pot. Cover and cook on low for 6 hours, enjoy!

NUTRITION:

Calories: 282	Fat: 12g	Carbs: 7g	Protein: 34g

Coconut Almond Cake

Serves: 6

INGREDIENTS:

- ➢ 1/2 cup coconut oil
- ➢ 2 teaspoons powdered stevia
- ➢ 2 large eggs
- ➢ 1 teaspoon vanilla extract
- ➢ 1 teaspoon almond extract
- ➢ 3/4 cup almond flour
- ➢ 3/4 cup coconut flour

INSTRUCTIONS:

Add all ingredients to a bowl and mix well everything is combined and there are no lumps. Turn your slow cooker on high and spray well with nonstick cooking spray. Pour your cake mixture into your slow cooker and insure, place on cover, and cook for about an hour, until a toothpick comes out clean when you insert it, enjoy!

NUTRITION:

Calories: 244	Fat: 20g	Carbs: 11g	Protein: 7g

I hope you enjoyed this book and found the nutritional information of value and the recipes easy to complete and delicious. If you did find the book of value, please go back over to Amazon and post a four or five star review. If you have any concerns, suggestions or questions about the content, please send me an email and I will do my best to resolve your concerns or answer your questions.

Get Fit, Stay Fit !
Jesse – Jesse@fitrecipe.net

38370684R00044

Made in the USA
San Bernardino, CA
04 September 2016